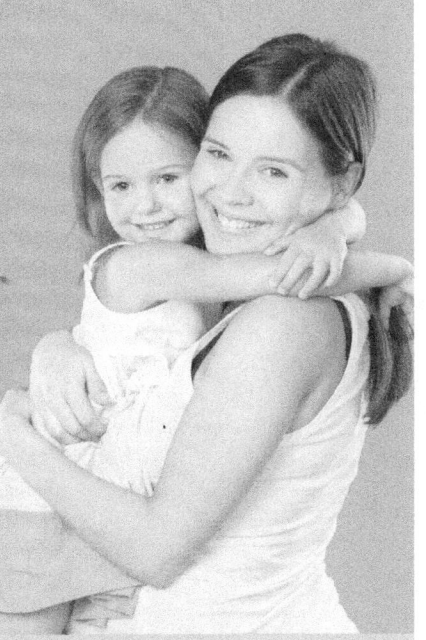

MOMS WITH ADHD

Strategies for Women Parenting With Adult ADHD

Moms With ADHD:

Strategies for Women Parenting With Adult ADHD

Kristen Thrasher

© **Copyright Kristen Thrasher 2022 - All rights reserved.**

The content contained within this book may not be reproduced, duplicated or transmitted without direct written permission from the author or the publisher. Under no circumstances will any blame or legal responsibility be held against the publisher, or author, for any damages, reparation, or monetary loss due to the information contained within this book. Either directly or indirectly. You are responsible for your own choices, actions, and results.

Legal Notice:

This book is copyright protected. This book is only for personal use. You cannot amend, distribute, sell, use, quote or paraphrase any part, or the content within this book, without the consent of the author or publisher.

Disclaimer Notice:

Please note the information contained within this document is for educational and entertainment purposes only. All effort has been executed to present accurate, up-to-date, and reliable, complete information. No warranties of any kind are declared or implied. Readers acknowledge that the author is not engaging in the rendering of legal, financial, medical, or professional advice. The content within this book has been derived from various sources. Please consult a licensed professional before attempting any techniques outlined in this book.

By reading this document, the reader agrees that under no circumstances is the author responsible for any losses, direct or indirect, which are incurred as a result of the use of the information contained within this document, including, but not limited to, — errors, omissions, or inaccuracies.

Table of Contents

Introduction

Chapter 1: The Surprising Amount of Moms With ADHD

Chapter 2: What it Feels Like Parenting With ADHD

Chapter 3: When Both Mom and Child Have ADHD

Chapter 4: Do's and Don'ts of Parenting with ADHD

Chapter 5: Strategies for Moms with ADHD

Chapter 6: Supporting Moms with ADHD

Conclusion

Introduction

Many mothers only learn they have been living with ADHD after their child begins to have symptoms. Once the parent addresses the diagnosis with the child, the mother will often realize that she has been living with the same exact symptoms for her entire life too. The mother will then be diagnosed with the condition herself.

Attention deficit hyperactivity disorder (ADHD) is a common childhood disorder, however boys are twice as likely to be diagnosed than girls. And not at all because boys are more susceptible, but rather because their symptoms tend to be more hyperactive-impulsive, which makes them much more noticeable than girls' symptoms.

Girls, on the other hand, often have symptoms of inattentiveness which causes no noticeable disturbances in their surroundings. This is why their condition most often goes overlooked, often into adulthood.

Because these symptoms never magically disappear in adulthood, many women are left undiagnosed, which leaves many women who unknowingly live with a condition that can affect every single aspect of their lives, including motherhood.

The problem for women is, by adulthood their ADHD symptoms are far greater while their ability to cope becomes much more difficult. Diagnosing and treating ADHD in adults can be lifesaving, however, as the condition affects more than 4 percent of adults in the United States.

Most women affected with adult ADHD also have at least one comorbid condition, such as anxiety, bipolar disorder, tics, depression, substance abuse, or learning disorders. In fact, a study of adult ADHD in the United States found a significantly higher proportion of females than males with ADHD receive treatment for substance abuse and mental problems.

While only about 12 percent of adult women with ADHD actually get treatment for the condition, it is very important to get treatment as early as possible. Women need to educate themselves about ADHD, particularly related to adulthood and motherhood. If a woman is struggling with disorganization, restlessness, focusing, and other similar issues, she should consult a medical professional to seek a diagnosis and seek medical care options. It is absolutely critical to treat the root issue.

There are several other symptoms women should be on the lookout for, including deflated self-esteem, drug and/or alcohol abuse, poor impulse control, mood difficulties, and excessive anxiety.

Treatment most often consists of medication with or without stimulants in an effort to strengthen the working memory, reduce distractibility, and enhance organizational ability, among many other things. However, treatment can be life-altering.

In fact, most women often speak of regret for not seeking help sooner. They also mention sadness or blame towards their parents for not getting them help earlier in life, as they are finally in control of their lives for the very first time as an adult.

In this book, we are going to take a look at exactly what parenting with ADHD looks like, specifically for moms who have ADHD. The chapters will be broken down as such: The Surprising Amount of Moms Who Have ADHD, What It Feels Like Parenting With ADHD, When Both Mom and Child Have ADHD, Do's and Don'ts of Parenting With ADHD, Strategies for Moms With ADHD, and Support for Moms With ADHD.

By the end of the book, you will have a better understanding of what ADHD in adulthood looks like, particularly related to motherhood. You will understand why so many women go undiagnosed until adulthood and the key symptoms to be on the lookout for if you think you yourself or a loved one might have ADHD.

You will also learn what to do when both you and your children have ADHD. There will be an entire chapter on several different do's and don'ts of parenting when either the parent or the child has ADHD, as well as an entire chapter with 25 different strategies for moms who have ADHD. Then, finally, there is a chapter with several different ways you can support your mom friends who have ADHD.

There is truly something inside this book for everyone, whether you have ADHD or you have a close friend, family member, or even a spouse or has ADHD. Without further odu, let's get started.

Chapter 1: The Surprising Amount of Moms Who Suffer With ADHD

The majority of women do not simply outgrow the ADHD symptoms they had when they were young girls. And, due to this, as adults they will often suffer from poor self-image, have a hard time with social obligations and relationships, and an inability to organize and complete tasks in a timely manner.

Women with ADHD are also more at risk for underachieving, being less successful than their peers, and are often scattered with things in life. Many women with ADHD may have also had either multiple jobs or career changes, often simply due to boredom.

More often than not, women with untreated ADHD find themselves struggling with parenting. Some moms may be a little more stressed with trying to deal with the structures that often come along with motherhood, depending on the age of their children. Many often find it overwhelming to try to keep things planned and managed. Women with untreated ADHD may also often feel as if they are "all over the place" and then become down on themselves for not feeling adequate as a mom.

These women also tend to have short-fused or reactive emotions, which means their frustration tolerance is lower, which leads to impatience and outbursts with their children. Many women have to function both at home with their children and in the workplace simultaneously. These responsibilities require very different skill sets along with frustration tolerance in order to stay on task without outbursts or abandoning the task before them.

Added stressors can make things even worse. Stay-at-home orders during the coronavirus pandemic challenged the ADHD-riddled working mom, for example, as they're expected to homeschool their children. Disorganization diminishes their ability to help with schoolwork or even teach their children organization skills. While poor time management leads to chronic tardiness and will often provoke anxiety in the child. Also, distractibility leads to poor task completion and unreliability.

Let's take a look at some statistics of ADHD in adults. ADHD among adults in 2001-2003, according to a Harvard Medical School, was 4.4% in the United States. However, the rate of ADHD in adults is likely underreported because as much as 85% of children with ADHD will likely still have the disorder as adults.

The diagnosis of ADHD among adults is actually growing four times faster than the ADHD diagnoses among children in the United States. Let's look at statistics for specific age groups.

- Ages 18-24: 4.5%
- Ages 25-34: 3.8%
- Ages 35-44: 4.6%

As research suggests, the majority of children with ADHD will also have ADHD as adults. A critical thing for children to learn is how to manage their ADHD symptoms. This may very well have a positive impact on their adult symptoms and whether or not their ADHD reaches into adulthood.

Many adults have since described experiencing milder symptoms and less impairments in functioning because they have learned their triggers in their childhood as well as specific ways to cope with their ADHD symptoms.

Some adults have even learned to cope with their symptoms so well that they no longer meet the criteria for an ADHD diagnosis in adulthood, although they were diagnosed as a child. For clarity, they may still have some of the ADHD symptoms, but not enough to receive an actual diagnosis.

Most research suggests that ADHD never truly goes away. However, some adults do report less symptoms. For example, hyperactivity symptoms do typically decline and decrease with maturity and age. Only 11% of adults with ADHD actually receive any kind of ADHD treatment, whether it is medication or behavioral therapy.

What's more, some women may go undiagnosed and therefore remain untreated due to co-occuring mental health conditions that will actually mask the symptoms of their ADHD. Let's take a look at some of these conditions below, as well as their percentages.

- Impulse controle: 20%
- Anxiety disorder: 47%
- Substance abuse disorder: 15%
- Mood disorder: 38%

While you can clearly see the abundance of women who have ADHD, you can also now see why so many remain undiagnosed. Because of the amount of women who remain undiagnosed and, therefore, untreated, it is fair to say that these numbers simply cannot be completely accurate. Which leads researchers to believe there are many, many more women who have adult ADHD than the numbers actually show.

Chapter 2: Parenting with ADHD

Almost all new parents suffer from the same symptoms that could fall under a diagnosis of ADHD, including forgetfulness, losing important items, lack of focus on directions, disorganization, and a general sense of foggy thinking.

The simple act of adding a fully dependent tiny human being to your busy schedule is bound to cause these things. The lack of sleep can easily be attributed to the new baby. However, if these symptoms continue as your child grows and you are getting more rest, instead of decreasing, it may be that ADHD is present and has simply been undiagnosed.

In fact, the first little signs of ADHD may not be fully present until certain life circumstances begin to overwhelm you, such as taking on huge responsibilities such as a new job, marriage, or even becoming a parent yourself. This is often when your former precocious ways of coping are suddenly no longer enough for the exhausting new challenges in your life.

Those with ADHD often find that doubling their workload makes hiding, coping, or even denying their symptoms to be virtually impossible, even after years and years of somehow managing to stay on course. When you realize you have made the switch from "normal chaos" to something much deeper, or "out-of-control chaos", the first step should be talking to your medical professional about your symptoms. Your medical professional will be able to offer medication or therapy techniques to help increase your focus and simultaneously ease your symptoms.

Did you know that if you have a child with ADHD, that there is actually a 60 percent chance that either you or your child's other parent also has ADHD? It is not always the dad, either. Research has shown that there is actually a 50/50 chance that the mother of the child with ADHD will also have ADHD herself.

While this may surprise you because ADHD is often missed in both girls and women, that doesn't mean it is not present. In fact, quite the opposite is true. What's worse, overlooking ADHD in women seems to only cause more problems because most women who have ADHD also have some other conditions along with it, such as anxiety or depression. While treating these side conditions might help them feel better temporarily, it will never fully cure the root of their underlying problems, which are the ADHD symptoms.

Moms with adult ADHD often have it twice as hard as moms who do not have ADHD - it is no easy task trying to balance your personal life, family, and your career while battling attention deficit hyperactivity disorder. Being a mom is a hard job, whether you are a busy professional trying to balance kids, a career, and everything else, or you are a stay-at-home mom which has plenty of challenges of its own. Whichever category you fall under, it's much more difficult when you're a mom with ADHD.

There are a plethora of ADHD medications now available for women; however, many of these medicines do not make it through the entire day. And, the reality is, most women are still the primary caregivers. After an exhausting day at work, moms with ADHD are still expected to motivate others, organize activities, prepare meals, and pay bills, as well as other household chores, none of which are easy for the ADHD-mind.

Many psychologists have found that mothers will often go to any lengths to find help for their child with ADHD, but leave her own ADHD needs unmet. However, ADHD must be addressed as a "family issue" rather than a "child issue" when the mother also has ADHD. Supporting the mother's needs as well becomes a crucial part of helping the child who also has ADHD, if not just as important.

However, the sad reality is, few women get the help and support they truly need. Husbands likely do not understand what they could be doing to help their wives and may simultaneously have unrealistic expectations of both the responsibilities as well as the relationship.

There are also few support groups that focus on the unique needs of moms with ADHD. Other family members, especially in-laws, may even criticize the way the house looks, or other obvious signs of the problems due to ADHD symptoms.

You do not have to be super-mom! Accept that you have ADHD. As women, we tend to overlook our own needs, because we are so accustomed to tending to the needs of others. It becomes hard to admit that you can't do it all, aren't absolutely perfect, and might actually need help. The best thing you can do for yourself is to get out of denial, and simply accept that you have ADHD. Then, figure out what to do next.

A great way to simplify your life is to ask other family members for help. This helps you tremendously, while also teaches you responsibility at the same time, because this delegation includes solving problems together. Families work best when they work together as a team. Have your family do the tasks that aren't your favorite and stick with the tasks that you enjoy and are able to do well.

Always remember: having ADHD does NOT make you a bad mother! In fact, quite the opposite is true! It gives you the ability to create a loving, nurturing, and exciting home for you and your family, while empathizing with your children and coming up with creative solutions to life's many problems.

Rather than focusing on the negative aspects, focus on minimizing the weaknesses of ADHD and, instead, learn to appreciate the gifts it brings. Because your kids won't remember that your floors weren't perfectly swept and mopped, but they will always remember how much you loved them.

Below are some helpful tips for moms with ADHD:

- Learn communication strategies
- Have family meetings
- Explain your ADHD symptoms to your family
- Keep a calendar and use different colored inks for different schedules
- Schedule down time to re-energize
- Solve problems together, instead of pointing fingers
- Pick your battles
- Work together as a team
- Take time to cool down before getting into a heated family argument
- Get professional help with managing kids who have ADHD
- Establish quiet times/zones
- Create routines
- Keep explanations short

- Don't fight with picky eaters- instead use vitamins and healthy snacks
- Be flexible
- Get your partner to take over when you feel yourself start to lose it
- Hire a sitter when you're working on something at home
- Be consistent - even if it is difficult
- Take time away together with your spouse
- Find humor in the little things
- Get outside help for chores that create tension in your relationships
- Problem solve ahead of time
- Do all you can the night before to avoid morning chaos
- Create the no interruptions rule at the dinner table

Chapter 3: When Both Mom and Child Have ADHD

A story we regularly hear is a child being diagnosed with ADHD only for his or her mother to recognize the symptoms and realize that she herself has the disorder as well.

While it is often a surprise to the mother, it is not much of a surprise whatsoever to the medical professional, as they know ADHD is highly hereditary. In fact, 25 percent of parents of kids they diagnose are going to have it.

It also doesn't come as a surprise to most medical professionals that many mothers who meet the criteria for ADHD haven't been diagnosed and don't have a clue they themselves have the condition as well. There is still a lot of stigma and lack of understanding surrounding adults with ADHD, as sad as this may be.

Mothers with undiagnosed ADHD often find themselves extremely overwhelmed by the demands of parenting and often struggle to meet the needs of their children. They often find it hard to keep up with their children's schedules as they lack the organizational skills, and often even find it very stressful to manage their children's behaviors.

The majority of mothers are more likely to be diagnosed and treated for depression rather than ADHD. Which is unfortunate as treating the ADHD, which is their underlying problem, would benefit both the children and the mother greatly.

Research has shown that intervention for children with ADHD tends to be less effective when a primary caretaker parent also has ADHD, as medication treatment requires a lot of parental organization in order to deal with the insurance, make the doctor's appointments, fill the prescriptions, and then, finally, ensure the child takes the medicine while monitoring the side effects. The child's treatment will be less effective if their treatment regimen is not consistent.

There are a number of studies that actually look specifically at parent training, and the biggest predictor of treatment being less effective for children, is when a parent also has ADHD. In fact, all across the board, behavioral treatment for children with ADHD is simply less effective when one or both parents also have ADHD.

It is most common for mothers to discover that they have ADHD that was not diagnosed when they were children. This is because of the way ADHD presents itself so differently in the two genders. While men tend to have hyperactive forms of ADHD, women tend to have the inattentive and/or impulsive forms of ADHD instead.

These women may have been chronically underachieving and disorganized back in grade school, but since they are often not as disruptive as boys were, they were, more often than not, simply overlooked.

Now, we see moms who are being pulled between all kinds of things in their family and work life, and seem to be extremely stressed out. However, we most often tend to automatically think of either depression or anxiety. This is because we seem to associate depression and anxiety more with women, instead of seeing ADHD, which is the underlying deficit, which makes it so difficult to manage all of those things.

Getting a diagnosis itself can help alleviate stress and reduce guilt for a mother who has ADHD. The majority of women with ADHD simply don't realize they actually have ADHD, and are therefore untreated.

Many women realize they struggled in school, and perhaps even at work, in their marriage, and raising their children, but they simply cannot seem to understand why this is so. They will become frustrated and even demoralized. Rather than blaming themselves and believing they are failing, with an ADHD diagnosis, they will be able to understand that they have a genetic disorder as their child does.

Treatment for ADHD can vastly improve a mother's parenting skills, while also reducing stress for the entire family. ADHD treatment often involves stimulant medication; however, it may also include behavioral therapy. With proper treatment, a mother will be able to give her kids more focused attention while also becoming better organized herself.

However, after finding a working treatment regimen, mothers often report they all of a sudden feel less overwhelmed and are finally able to be more comfortable and relaxed with their children.

One of the big challenges of parenting children with ADHD is that these children will often have mild to extreme behavior problems. They are more prone to outbursts and tantrums when things don't go their way, and also have very low frustration tolerances. It is very difficult for all parents to respond effectively to this kind of behavior, but even more so for mothers who have ADHD themselves as well.

In order to manage your ADHD child's behavior successfully, mothers must remain calm and consistent, while keeping their own emotions out of the equation. Mothers need to avoid reacting emotionally to behaviors that are problematic and pay close attention to and respond positively to behaviors they want to encourage. However, none of these things are easy if you suffer from adult ADHD.

Research shows that when mothers get treatment for their own ADHD, their behavior management skills actually improve, which leads to an increase in positive parent-child interactions and more effective direction for their children. Therefore, treating the mother's ADHD <u>first</u> may be extremely important in helping the child overcome their own behavior problems.

There is, however, a shortage of medical professionals who feel comfortable both diagnosing and treating adults with ADHD. ADHD is similar to where depression was 20-something years ago, where it was something that only psychiatrists treated, before becoming primary care, and then finally becoming something that primary care doctors routinely screen for. Whereas ADHD is very common, it is still seldom screened for in adults, as it equally should be, just as depression and multiple other conditions are.

Medical professionals do not get near as much training in diagnosing and prescribing stimulant medications for ADHD as they do diagnosing and prescribing antidepressants for depression. Many medical professionals also worry about the potential for abusing stimulant medications, which can make them feel uncomfortable even prescribing them. Which is another reason many medical professionals often steer clear of an ADHD diagnosis and stay more in the anxiety and depression realm.

What's more, many organizations that treat children with ADHD are leary about including parents in their coverage. Family medicine should be a place that should work for the entire family, not just the children. However, due to the discomfort with using stimulants, many adults are more likely to be prescribed an antidepressant instead.

40

Chapter 4: Do's and Don'ts of Parenting with ADHD

There is a very high likelihood if you have ADHD, one or more of your children do too. Depending on the severity and type of your child's symptoms, household routines and normal rule-making can become almost impossible, which means you will need to adopt different approaches. It can be very frustrating to cope with some of the behaviors which result from your child's ADHD, but there are several ways to make your life easier.

As a mom, you must first accept the fact that your child with ADHD has a functionally different brain from that of a non-ADHD child. Children with ADHD are still able to learn what is and what is not acceptable, however ADHD does make them more prone to impulsive behavior.

You will likely need to modify your behavior in order to learn how to manage the behavior of your ADHD child. While medication may be the first step in managing your child's symptoms, there are also several behavioral techniques that can help manage ADHD symptoms. By following the guidelines below, you can limit destructive behavior and help your child overcome self-doubt.

There are two basic principles of behavior management therapy. The first is known as punishment, which is removing rewards by following bad behavior with appropriate consequences, leading to the extinguishing of bad behavior. The second is known as positive reinforcement, which is rewarding and encouraging good behavior.

By using these forms of behavior management therapy, you will teach your child to understand that actions have consequences by establishing rules and clear outcomes for following or disobeying these rules. In order for this to work properly, you must decide ahead of time which behaviors are appropriate and which are not.

The goal of this behavioral modification is to help your child understand the consequences of an action and learn to control his or her impulse to act on it. This requires affection, patience, strength, empathy, and energy on the part of the mom. You must first decide which behaviors you will and will not tolerate. It is very crucial that you stick to these guidelines. To be inconsistent and choose to allow the behavior one day and punish the same behavior the next day, is extremely harmful to a child's improvement.

While it is important to clearly define the rules, it is also important to allow <u>some</u> flexibility. Although it is good to consistently reward good behaviors while discouraging destructive ones, you shouldn't be too strict with your children. Children with ADHD may not adapt to change as well as others. Your child should be allowed to make mistakes as they are learning the rules.

Odd behaviors that aren't detrimental to your child, or anyone else, should be accepted as part of your child's individual personality. Please understand that it is actually harmful to discourage your child's "quirky" behaviors just because you believe they are unusual.

A common problem from children with ADHD can be aggressive outbursts. Believe it or not, an effective way to calm both you and your overactive child can be an old-fashioned "time-out", which should be explained as a period of time for your child to calm down and think about the negative behavior they have displayed. Remember, try to ignore mildly disruptive behaviors, as these are a good way for your child to release their built up energy. However, abusive, destructive, or intentionally disruptive behavior that absolutely goes against the rules you have already established, should always be punished.

Let's look at some good strategies below to adopt in your life to make it easier when you are a mom with ADHD raising children with ADHD below.

Organize and simplify your children's lives

In order to allow your children to take a break from the chaos of everyday life, create a quiet and special place for them to read and do their homework. Make every effort to reduce unnecessary distractions and to help your children know where everything goes. You should also always keep your home neat, clean and organized to give your children a sense of peace and calmness.

Structure is your friend

Create a structured routine for your children, and make sure you stick with it each and every day. Establish different routines for different areas in your children's life, such as playtime, mealtime, homework, and bedtime. You can provide essential structure for your child even with the most mundane of tasks, such as having your child lay out his or her clothes for the next day or pack the backpack the night before school.

Regulate sleep patterns

Bedtime tends to be a difficult thing for children who have ADHD. However, a lack of sleep only makes several ADHD symptoms worse, such as recklessness, hyperactivity, and inattention. It is important that your child gets the proper amount of sleep. In order to ensure they get enough sleep, cut out stimulants like caffeine and sugar, and decrease television time. Also, a calming bedtime routine.

Limit distractions

Children who have ADHD are more prone to be easily distracted, there is absolutely no way around it. For this reason, the television, computer, and video games should be regulated and limited by adult supervision. In fact, by increasing time doing engaging activities outside your home, and decreasing time with electronics, your child will have an outlet for all of their built-up energy.

It is okay to take a break.

It is absolutely normal to become frustrated or overwhelmed with both yourself and your child from time to time. You simply can't be supportive ALL the time. Just as your child will need to take breaks while studying, you may very well need your own breaks for your sanity as well. Scheduling alone time is important for any mother. Some good options include:

- Hiring a babysitter
- Going for a walk
- Taking a relaxing bath
- Exercising at the gym

Encourage out-loud thinking

A lot of children with ADHD lack self-control, which causes them to both act and talk without thinking. It is very important to try to understand your child's thought process in order to help him rectify impulsive behaviors. Try asking your child to verbalize their thoughts and reasoning when the urge to act out arises.

Divide your tasks up into smaller tasks

Use a wall calendar to remind your children of their duties. Begin with color coding your children's different chores, activities, and even homework assignments in order to keep them from becoming overwhelmed with their everyday responsibilities. Their morning routines should even be broken down into smaller, concrete tasks, so that nothing is left to question and everyone knows exactly what to do and what time without becoming overwhelmed.

Encourage your child to get enough exercise

Physical activity helps a child focus their attention on specific movements, which may decrease impulsivity. Exercise also burns excess energy in healthy ways and helps to improve concentration while decreasing the risk for depression and anxiety, as well as stimulating the brain in healthy ways. In fact, many professional athletes have ADHD. Experts actually believe that sports can help a child who has ADHD find a constructive way to focus their energy and attention, as well as their passion.

Calm yourself down first

If you are aggravated, it will be nearly impossible to calm your impulsive or overactive children. However, children tend to mimic the behaviors they see around them, causing them to remain composed and controlled if you do. Particularly try keeping your cool during an outburst, and watch and see what they do. Take time to relax, collect your thoughts, and breathe before attempting to calm your child down. Remember, the more calm you are, the more calm your child will become too.

Believe in your children

Believe it or not, your child is not meaning to cause you stress, and likely doesn't even realize the stress that their condition can cause. Which is why it is so important to remain positive and encouraging, even when you feel as if you have reached your limits. Always try to praise your child's positive behavior so they know when they have done something right. Always have confidence in your child and their future, no matter how many ADHD symptoms they are showing in the here and now. It is very likely they will outgrow some, or even all, of their symptoms as they enter adulthood.

Find specialized and individualized counseling for your child

You were not made to do everything. While your child certainly needs your encouragement, they also need professional help. A professional therapist can be a great way to provide another outlet for your child, so please do not be afraid to ask for help when you feel your child needs it. Many mothers become so hyper-focused on their children that they will neglect their own mental needs. A therapist will help manage your child's anxiety and stress, but can also help manage your own as well.

We wouldn't be able to have a list of "do's" if we didn't have a list of "don'ts" to follow. You will notice that this list is much shorter than the previous list. However, it is important to still note a few things. Let's look at a few don'ts below.

Don't get overwhelmed and lash out

Never forget that your child's misbehavior is caused by a disorder. While ADHD may not be visible on the outside, it is still a disability, and should be treated as such. Remember that your child can't just be "normal" or "snap out of it" when you begin to get angry or frustrated and cut them some slack instead of lashing out.

Don't sweat the small stuff

Always be willing to make compromises with your child. For instance, if she has accomplished two or three of the chores you have assigned, consider being flexible with the third, uncompleted task, rather than making her finish it every single time. This is a learning process where even small steps count and can be monumentale for your child.

Don't ever let the disorder or your child take control

Be nurturing and patient, but don't allow yourself to be bullied or intimidated by your child's behaviors. Always remember that you establish the rules and acceptable behaviors in your home because you are the parent.

Don't be negative

Remember, what is embarrassing or stressful today, will fade away with tomorrow. While it sounds simplistic, always take things one day at a time and keep everything in perspective. Try to always remain positive instead of negative. For every bad day your child has, there has to be a good day in there as well.

Chapter 5: Strategies for Moms with ADHD

I would like to personally give you a standing ovation if you are a mother with ADHD who is raising one or more children who also have ADHD. You don't need me to tell you that you have your hands full. As a mom with ADHD, the challenges of parenting a child with ADHD seem to only multiply.

It will often seem like the entire deck is stacked against you. Because girls most commonly have the inattentive form of ADHD, and often don't get diagnosed until adulthood, women are most always diagnosed later in life than men.

In fact, many moms only discover they have ADHD while having their children evaluated for the disorder. Their child's symptoms are all too familiar. They will then often seek an assessment for themselves as well. Most women with ADHD are actually diagnosed with another disorder before getting the accurate ADHD diagnosis.

The trouble doesn't end there, however, as there are many obstacles to overcome after being officially diagnosed. Most mothers will put themselves last when it comes to health care, especially mental health, while often taking on the majority of child care. Women who suffer from chronic stress, such as that caused by ADHD symptoms, are actually more at risk for stress-related conditions.

In this chapter, I would like to go over some strategies that I have found helpful as a mom myself suffering with adult ADHD.

Don't stop what you are currently doing.

You will often begin a task, then abandon it to move on for another task, when you suddenly remember it needs to be done. However, then yet another task runs across your mind. Does this sound familiar to you? This is one of the worst habits that will always steer you off track. Always complete one task before moving on to the next. Hint: write down the other tasks you remember, while in the middle of the original task, so that you can remember it later.

Use visual cues or reminders.

Color-code items to make them easy to spot and unlikely to be mistaken for someone else's. You can even differentiate toothbrushes by using different colors to prevent confusion and swapping unsanitary oral hygiene during the morning rush.

Start your day off slowly.

Create the habit of always setting your alarm and getting up at least 15-20 minutes earlier than you need to get up. Then use these extra precious minutes for gathering your thoughts, meditating, and going over your to-do list for the day.

Post everyone's schedules.

Create a calendar for each upcoming week, and then place it in a location where everyone can see it. Make sure it is color-coded so that, even at a glance, everyone will know what everyone else is doing and where they are going to be at what times and on what specific days. Fewer surprises means fewer misunderstandings and fewer moments of embarrassment, disrupted activities, and frayed nerves.

Make recordings.

Instead of nagging your children every morning with the same phrases, make a tape recording about what needs to be done. For instance, specific tape recordings for certain times and routines, such as the mornings before school. It could be something as simple as, "Brush your teeth, my darlings, get dressed, eat your breakfast, and don't forget to go potty and grab a jacket on your way out the door." You could even have your children make their own recordings so they hear their voices telling themselves what to do each morning.

Be flexible, especially at meal times.

Deciding what to serve for dinner is a chore in and of itself. Don't give yourself a heart attack by forcing your children to sit down at the table at dinnertime. If they are hyperactive (which, odds are, if you are ADHD, your children are also), let them lie on the floor, stand up, or even sprawl out on a chair. This will ensure meal times to be more relaxing for everyone, and your children will probably even eat more because of this.

Even when you are home, hire a sitter sometimes.

If your children are hyperactive, a college student, or even a high-school student, can act as a support system. Student sitters will have the energy needed to keep up with and entertain an energized child, especially if you have the inattentive type of ADHD and become overwhelmed by an overactive home.

Take care of yourself first.

If you don't take care of yourself first, you will not be able to properly take care of your children. You must address your needs first so that you can better address the needs of your family and your children. Extensive research has shown that the most effective therapies to help treat the symptoms of ADHD are exercise, sleep hygiene, and mindfulness. In fact, taking proper care of yourself, will even put you in the right mindset to take care of your loved ones.

Make an obstacle course for yourself.

Before bedtime at night, find all of the items that you will need for the next day, such as your keys, briefcase, letters to be mailed, to-do list, grocery list, and whatever else you might need. Place them on a chair right in front of the door you normally exit in the mornings, so that it will literally block your path out of the house. Another idea is to place all of your must-have items in a basket and hang it at eye level by the exit door. Make sure to tie the other end of the hanger string to the doorknob so you will literally have to move the basket before opening the door. Both of these options are a fool-proof way to make sure you do not forget all of your must-have necessities for the day.

Give yourself more time.

When you have easily distractible family members, it is even more difficult to get everyone where they need to be on time. One way to help get you or your kids to where they need to go on time is to simply start getting ready earlier. When you need to be somewhere, try starting getting ready at least 15-20 minutes earlier than you think you need. This will prevent you from rushing around and getting frantic or forgetting something. Start the kids moving earlier too.

Don't make promises you can't keep.

Promises are often hard to keep, and life is chaotic enough without making empty promises that you will have to fall short on. The closest you should EVER come to making a promise is to simply say, "We will see how it goes." Never lock yourself into things, because you never know what might happen that will cause you to have to cancel your plans. However, if the opportunity arises, go ahead and offer a pleasant surprise.

Pause before making big decisions.

Because of ADHD, you probably have a tendency to think and act impulsively. This will often lead to negative consequences, especially when it comes to making emotional or significant parenting decisions. Always take a pause before making an important parenting decision. Try to find a quiet place away from your children, and the phone, in order to have the time to do some deep breathing and allow yourself to think through both the positive and negative aspects before making your final decision.

Ask for social support.

Due to the many challenges of living with adult ADHD, many moms find they have difficulty with social skills, relationships, and even self-esteem. Talking with someone who understands what you are going through, especially hearing about how others deal with these same issues, will make a big difference in how you are able to cope with your condition. Talk to your doctor about individual counseling or support groups if you find yourself struggling with these issues and it's affecting your family or home life.

Get a tutor.

Many moms who suffer with adult ADHD will not have the patience to help with homework, especially when their ADHD meds wear off around the same time as the child's. Instead of getting frustrated with yourself and your child, hire a high-school student a few days a week to help your child, and also take the pressure off yourself.

Create structure in your home

Setting up rules to maintain order in your house does not make you a buzzkill. Research shows that children, including teens, benefit and even actually thrive with structure. Because ADHD often runs in families, you are likely dealing with your child's inherited symptoms as well as your own. Therefore, structure is one of the main things you can count on as a tool to help everyone manage their ADHD symptoms.

Have the whole family help create the schedule.

Create a family council: it can be one of the most effective tools for dealing with your individual family challenges. Pick a set day each week to review schedules for the following week, noting any special arrangements or deviations from the normal routine. Encourage your children to participate and express their opinions, especially about particular events that will affect them, such as a movie they are dying to see or a family outing on the weekend. Then, as a family, you can create a master calendar for the upcoming week, based on everyone's input. This will also leave less room for surprises and upset children.

Take every day step by step.

Everyday tasks are often a challenge for moms who suffer from adult ADHD. you may find you are either forgetting to be places are always missing deadlines as having ADHD makes it hard to prioritize as well as focus. These exact things are often what lead many moms to have sudden mood swings, become impatient, and even have angry outbursts. Focus on being more patient with yourself, and explain to your family, including your children, how your ADHD affects you. Simply ask your loved ones for their understanding and patience. The most important thing to remember is to take your daily tasks one step at a time, concentrating on one task before you move on to the next item on your list.

Set firm routines.

Setting up firm routines that work for you to handle things such as meal planning, household chores, and homework checking, wil help you get AND stay organized while reducing the concentration required to get these things done daily.

Take a (much-needed) break after work.

Coming home to a full house of kids with ADHD, is overwhelming, to put it politely. Make sure to schedule down time into your post-work schedule, whether it's taking a short drive to a nearby ocean or lake, or driving through Starbucks on your way home. Do something that helps you to relax and ground yourself before you ever get home, so that you can be the best version of yourself for your children.

Stay in the game.

Come up with ways for your children to "pull you back" when they notice you become distracted or daydreaming. (It happens to even the best of us, especially those of us with inattentive ADHD.) Decide upon a "trigger" word or comment they can use, such as "Earth to mom!" This will serve as a reminder for you to regain your focus on what is most important - your children.

Don't try to do everything on your own

There is absolutely no reason you should ever try to do this thing called motherhood completely on your own. Seek out support from your family and friends. Simply knowing that you don't have to face parenting challenges alone, will help you cope with emotional and stress issues. A friend to talk with, carpools, and a work-out partner can all help ease the chaos and stress in your day-to-day life.

Become and stay organized.

Mom life is extremely busy, so getting and staying organized may currently be one of your biggest challenges. Mom's with ADHD don't make enough chemicals in the organizing center of the brain, making it harder on them than other people to keep things organized, remember details, and listen to instructions. However, there are so many different amazing calendars, apps, and other systems, you just need to find the right one for you and your family. An organizational life coach can also provide some great tailored tips to your lifestyle.

Pay attention

I know what you're thinking: "I can't focus because I have ADHD and I have a very low attention span." This is another way list-making can come to the rescue. Whenever someone tells you something you need to remember, make sure to either write it down or add it to your calendar with an alarm to remind you at the appropriate time. Don't hesitate to stop someone and day, "Hold on, let me write this down", or "Let me add that to my calendar". People love this because it shows you care enough about their needs to make a note and they won't mind waiting for you to do so.

Make lists

There are very few moms, with or without ADHD, that are equipped with organizational thinking that they don't need a written list. It's not only while children are small either, most of us will always need these details written down in some form or fashion. The activities schedule will most often continue to grow as your children's play dates change to sports events and games. It gets easier with multiple children, as after you have developed the perfect list for your first child, you simply have to tweak it with each new child. You can put your lists in multiple places, in fact, the more places the better, such as on the fridge, in your phone, or in your planner or calendar.

In conclusion, you just freed up some more "me time"!!! Because you will no longer have to reschedule appointments you missed or double back to fix the tasks you forgot about, you will now be able to schedule in some down time for yourself. Take a bubble bath, go for a walk, or grab a cup of coffee with a friend - you deserve it! Always schedule something that helps you feel refreshed every single day. It doesn't have to be a big chunk of time, but it needs to

be something that makes you feel like you, not a mom, but you. When you take care of yourself first, you will have enough energy to take care of your loved ones.

Chapter 6: Support for Moms with ADHD

The world we live in most commonly thinks of ADHD as a young, male disorder. However, millions of adults suffer from ADHD. The majority of those that get diagnosed as children have the hyperactive-impulsive form of ADHD. while those with the predominantly inattentive symptoms, such as difficulty paying attention to details, forgetfulness and trouble finishing tasks, difficulty focusing, and lack of organization, often go undiagnosed as children.

This is troublesome for women and girls, who are better able to mask their symptoms than males because their inattentive symptoms don't stand out as much as the male gender, as a whole.

The main thing many medical professionals see with women being treated with ADHD is a strong sense of overwhelm. Many moms with ADHD talk about things such as to-lists created but never used, persistent stacks of papers around the house, guilt and frustration because they can't seem to get it together, and uncontrollable emotions and feelings of inadequacy. In fact, many women with ADHD often admit to wondering how other women are able to do the simple things like cleaning the house, staying organized, or just moving from basic thought to action.

Parenting with ADHD presents a major challenge for women, as the majority of women are the household managers and also the primary parent. In fact, a lot of women with ADHD believe it is much easier to go to work all day than to be at home with their children for any length of time. This is because you lose the structure of your day when you are at home with your children.

To make matters worse, ADHD is genetic and tends to run in families. This means that moms with ADHD are more likely to have children with ADHD. If a woman suspects that she has ADHD, she should get an evaluation from a medical professional as soon as possible, specifically one with experience in adult ADHD. This evaluation should include a very intricate interview that reviews both past and current difficulties, including school performance, social relationships, and work history, as well as other medical or psychiatric conditions.

It takes someone really experienced to get to the bottom or root of the issue, otherwise you could easily wind up with a diagnosis or anxiety or depression. Anxiety and depression are both really common in women who have ADHD. Many medical professionals lack an understanding of exactly how ADHD can affect women, which often makes it difficult to get an accurate diagnosis.

Ultimately, after receiving an official diagnosis, you will need some support. Whether that is from a therapist, a support group, a spouse, or a close family member, it is very important to have that support. In this chapter, we are going to look at some things you can do to support a mom with ADHD.

Parenting is hard enough for adults without ADHD. However, for moms with ADHD, it is even more challenging. Disorganization, impulsiveness, forgetfulness, distractibility, and time perception, among other issues, make the tasks involved with running a household and parenting that much more difficult.

Below, let's look at five different things you can do to help support mom's who have ADHD.

Plan an outdoor activity

Plan any kind of outdoor activity, and then literally drag her out of the house if you have to. First, make sure she is not feeling overly stressed or burned out. Surprise her and her kids with a trip to the local pool or a day at the park. While she may be cranky at first, if you leave her alone and get her kids involved, she is likely to soon join in and thank you for the outing by the end of the day. You will have a great day out with your friend and she will enjoy a break from her regular life.

Tell her dinner is on you

Many women with ADHD have trouble keeping track of time, meaning dinner is often quick and late.

Treat her to a meal by sending over a pot roast with all the fixings, or another meal of your choice. You could even treat her entire family to a sit-down meal together. Then, don't forget to help with the dishes afterwards, or they are bound to sit in the sink for who knows how long. A stress-free dinner, and clean-up, is always, always appreciated.

Throw a folding party

The next time a mom friend tells you she needs to fold the laundry, head right on over there to help her. Trust me, it's likely already clean. Mom's with ADHD just aren't quite capable of the folding part. Bring the wine and stay there to prevent her from getting sidetracked. When she wanders into another room and begins talking about what needs to be done in there, kindly remind her you are there to help her get the laundry done today. Don't leave until every last bit of laundry is not just folded, but put away as well. You will have fun with your friend and help her accomplish something that she has been trying, and failing, to do on her own for weeks, or even months.

Schedule an errand day

Schedule time specifically to run errands so she can knock out some to-do list items or overdue errands. Have her keep a running list of any task that comes to mind and then use this list to plan a day in order to complete every item on her list. From hiring an electrician, to paying bills, you are there to keep her on track and make the day fun. Remember to keep the day light hearted and help eliminate any distractions.

Have an "I hate people day"

Sensory overload is common in women who have ADHD. After three to four weeks of having anxiety, depression, struggles with impulses, racing thoughts, inattention, and time management issues, they simply cannot handle much more. When that happens, they need a day of dim lights, books, movies, and thick blankets, or anything else that does not require a lot of brain power. Many women can't tolerate human interaction on these days beyond issuing simple groans or grunts on these days. Schedule an "I hate people day" for your friend, as she could probably use some downtime and will be well rested for the upcoming days ahead.

Conclusion

Moms with ADHD do most often have more on their plate than "normal" moms or moms who do not have children with ADHD; however, this seems to make them more stronger because of it. Because they have to be. They simply cannot give up and so they don't. They will take their child to medical professional after medical professional until finally getting to the root of the child's issues.

Which often leads most women to an ADHD diagnosis for herself as well. However, instead of her world being shaken by the news, it's like a fire comes alive inside of her instead. Because now, she finally knows the root of the majority of her problems. Where she may have been told all of her life she has bipolar, depression, or anxiety, and she may still have some of these issues, but now she knows the underlying issue, the ADHD.

She can then begin to plan and schedule her life, as well as her child's, around the ADHD diagnosis. So, no, it doesn't make moms weaker when they receive an ADHD diagnosis for themselves or their children, but rather, it only makes them stronger.

There are several do's and don'ts listed in this book as well as several strategies, both for moms with ADHD and for moms who have children with ADHD. There is even a section on how you can support your mom friends who have ADHD, as they could all use a little extra support.

Cut yourself some slack if your house is disorganized, if you lose track of time and show up late to your child's school, or if you can't find the bill you were supposed to mail last week - it's really NOT your fault. You are not just "spacey" or "out there". You have an actual condition that is causing these things. If you have several of the symptoms listed in this book, but have never received an official diagnosis, then you, too, might be one of the moms who are battling with untreated ADHD symptoms. Make the appointment with the medical professional to get the test to see if you qualify for an ADHD diagnosis.

    I promise it will only make your life easier if you do, not harder. Then you will know the exact steps to take next. You will know what medicines will help you instead of hurt you. You will know that it is not your fault. You will know which behavioral therapies will work best for you. You can create certain routines, schedules, and strategies to combat your symptoms and truly set yourself, and your child, up for the best shot at a "normal life".

Never let anyone look down on you because you have ADHD, especially if you are a mom. As you have seen in this book, motherhood is difficult alone, but add in the fact that if your child has ADHD it is highly likely that you yourself have ADHD as well, it makes being a mom that much more difficult. Instead of ever looking down on you, others should applaud you for getting up every single morning and giving it your best shot when the odds are clearly stacked against you.

Know that it is not your fault. You didn't ask for any of this, and neither did your child. Just as you give your child some slack and understand they cannot help some of their impulsive and disruptive behaviors, please understand that you cannot either. Your brain is simply wired differently. And that is a-okay. Because now you have this guide book filled with strategies and do's and don'ts to help you in your day-to-day life.

    As another mom with ADHD, raising a four-year-old son with ADHD, I have seen first hand the struggles we both have. I was not diagnosed with ADHD until adulthood. In fact, like many others, I didn't know much at all about ADHD until my son started showing ADHD symptoms. It was only then that I started to realize I had a lot of the same symptoms and acted in the same ways he did. I was impulsive. I was easily frustrated. I lost track of time. I struggled with organization and a hundred other things. And we fight, a lot. But, we also love each other, a lot. Because, at the end of the day, we share a common bond. And that is something that no one can ever take away.

I also have a six-year-old daughter who does not have ADHD. In fact, she is the complete opposite. She is the most relaxed, organized, and sweetest little girl in the whole world. I love both of my children equally even though they are night and day different. She almost never gets in trouble, and he has been known to throw one hell of a fit, in fact there was a time he seemed to be constantly throwing fits and screaming at me. But, I wouldn't change a single thing about each of them. They are both unique in their own ways, and while I do have to work more with him than I do with her, I wouldn't change a thing about my son.

I say all that to say that I have the best of both worlds. I have a child with ADHD and a child without ADHD. They honestly could not be any more opposite. They do fight occasionally. But they love each other fiercely, too. My son doesn't let anyone say a bad word about my daughter, and they are still so young. I am so excited to see how much their love continues to grow for each other as they grow up.

From one ADHD mom to another, I understand. When it feels like no one else understands, I do. And I am in your corner, rooting you on in every way. I wish you the very best. I know you can face whatever comes your way. And I am proud of you. Never give up. Take it each day at a time, one step at a time, until you find a routine you are happy with, and then stick with it! You've got this, girlfriend!

Other Books by Kristen Thrasher

87 Tips and Tricks for Women With ADHD: Survive the Chaos of Living With Adult ADHD, Manage Your Symptoms, and Live Your Best Life

301 Positive Affirmations for Adults Suffering With ADHD: For Women, Men, and Teens: Learn to Manage Your Impulsiveness, Hyperactivity, Irritability, Time Management, Disorganization, and More

ADHD in Adults: 2 Part Series: 87 Tips and Tricks for Women With ADHD and 301 Positive Affirmations for Adults Suffering With ADHD

Understanding ADHD in Women: Strategies for Women Diagnosed With ADHD in Adulthood: Manage

Your Symptoms as An Adult Living With Attention Deficit Hyperactivity Disorder

How ADHD Affects Relationships

Relationship Series: Gaslighting in Relationships and How ADHD Affects Relationships

Gaslighting in Relationships: Why Adults With ADHD are More Vulnerable to Gaslighting Specific Steps to Free Yourself From a Gaslit Relationship

Made in United States
North Haven, CT
14 June 2025